GET OUTDOORS

Go Hiking!

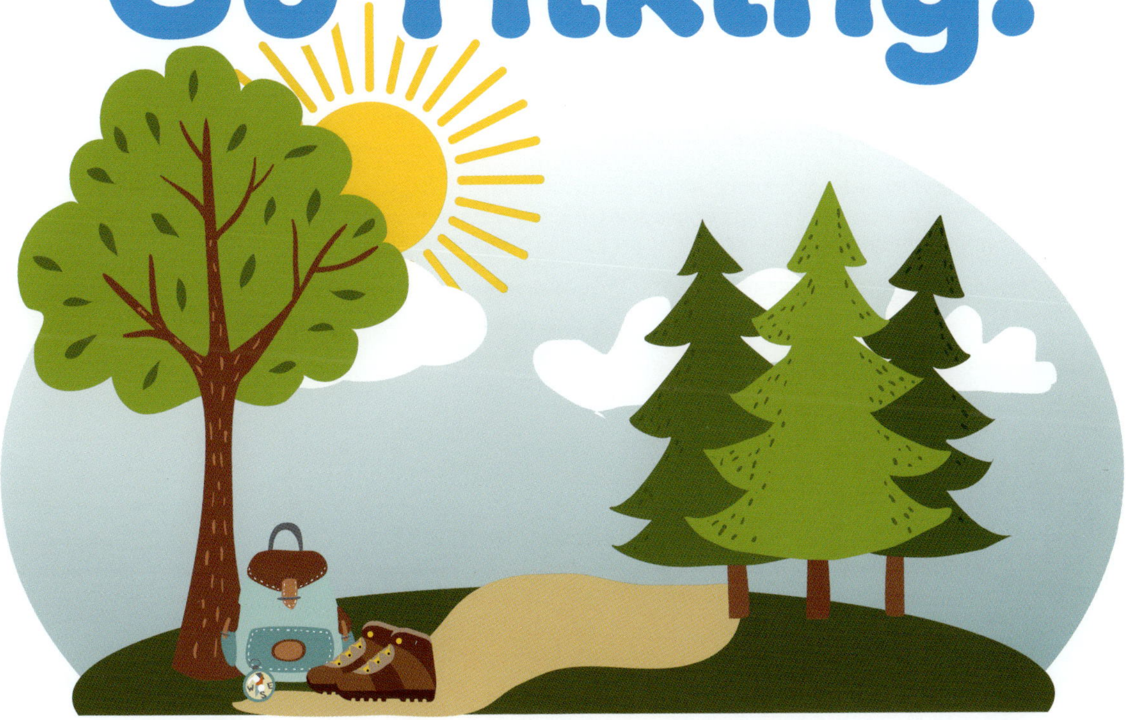

by Meghan Gottschall

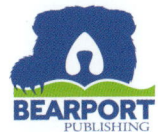
BEARPORT
PUBLISHING

Minneapolis, Minnesota

President: Jen Jenson
Director of Product Development: Spencer Brinker
Senior Editor: Allison Juda
Designer: Colin O'Dea

Library of Congress Cataloging-in-Publication Data

Names: Gottschall, Meghan, author.
Title: Go hiking! / by Meghan Gottschall.
Description: Fusion books. | Minneapolis, Minnesota : Bearport Publishing Company, [2022] | Series: Get outdoors | Includes bibliographical references and index.
Identifiers: LCCN 2021002674 (print) | LCCN 2021002675 (ebook) | ISBN 9781647479701 (library binding) | ISBN 9781647479770 (paperback) | ISBN 9781647479848 (ebook)
Subjects: LCSH: Hiking--Juvenile literature. | Outdoor recreation--Juvenile literature.
Classification: LCC GV199.52 .G68 2022 (print) | LCC GV199.52 (ebook) | DDC 796.51--dc23
LC record available at https://lccn.loc.gov/2021002674
LC ebook record available at https://lccn.loc.gov/2021002675

Copyright © 2022 Bearport Publishing Company. All rights reserved. No part of this publication may be reproduced in whole or in part, stored in any retrieval system, or transmitted in any form or by any means, electronic, mechanical, photocopying, recording, or otherwise, without written permission from the publisher.

For more information, write to Bearport Publishing, 5357 Penn Avenue South, Minneapolis, MN 55419. Printed in the United States of America.

Image Credits

Cover, © GraphicsRF.com/Shutterstock, © chuyuss/Shutterstock, © gresei/Shutterstock; 5, © Duangjai Manoonthamporn / EyeEm/Getty Images; 6, © 200degrees/Pixabay; 7T, © Sean Xu/Shutterstock; 7B, © Artarta/Shutterstock; 8, © THPStock/Shutterstock; 9, © AnnaStills/Shutterstock; 10, © Hsaart/Pixabay; 11, © Rawpixel.com/Shutterstock; 12L, © Luis Carlos Torres/Shutterstock; 12R, © chuyuss/Shutterstock; 13, © R.M. Nunes/Shutterstock; 14, © veronicabuffalo/Pixabay; 15, © rbkomar/Shutterstock; 17, © VP Photo Studio/Shutterstock; 18M, © PlumePloume/Pixabay; 18L, © wild wind/Shutterstock; 19, © Mauricio S Ferreira/Shutterstock; 20, © Marko Geber/Getty Images; 21, © Rick Nelson/Shutterstock; 23, © Sean Xu/Shutterstock; Background, © Clker-Free-Vector-Images/Pixabay, © Merggy/Shutterstock, © Shirstok/Shutterstock; Design elements, © Janjf93/Pixabay, © Kaliene/Pixabay, © aliaksei kruhlenia/Shutterstock, © NotionPic/Shutterstock, © JungleOutThere/Shutterstock, © Colorlife/Shutterstock, © Sudowoodo/Shutterstock

CONTENTS

A Hiking Adventure 4
Pick Your Path 6
What to Wear 8
Finding Your Way 10
Safety Gear 12
Hiking Snacks 14
On the Trail 16
Life in the Wild 18
Leave No Trace 20
Take a Hike. 22
Glossary 24
Index. 24

A HIKING ADVENTURE

Grab your backpack and your **compass**. We're going on a hike!

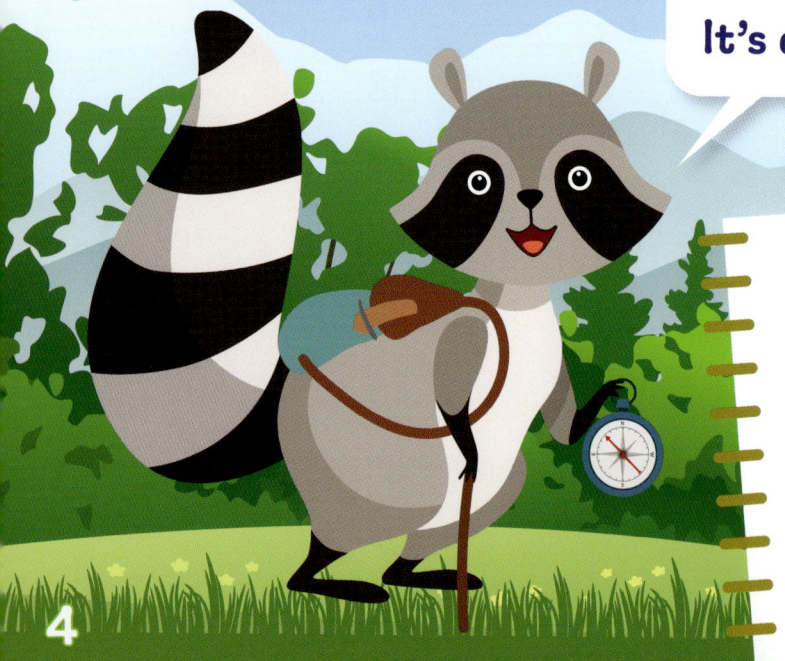

Hi, I'm Rory Raccoon, and I love to GET OUTDOORS! It's a beautiful day.

More than 45 million people go hiking in the United States every year.

A hike is a walk through nature. It's a great way to explore the outdoors. What will you see on your hike? Follow a trail and find out. Let's get started on our hiking adventure!

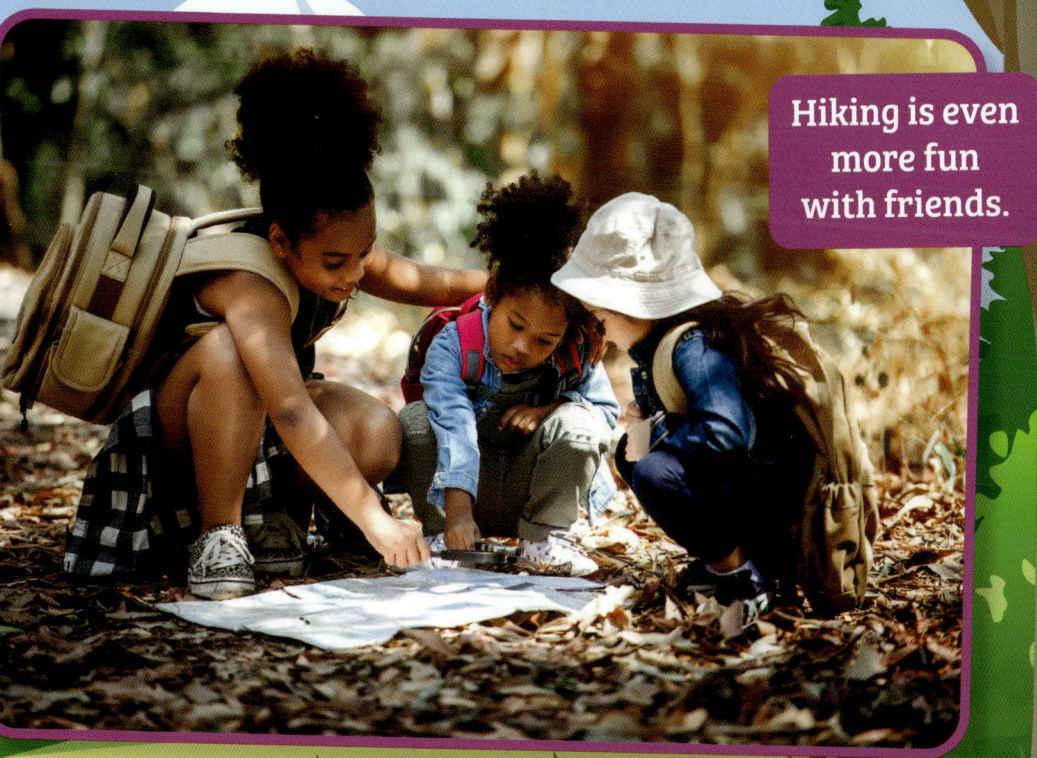

Hiking is even more fun with friends.

PICK YOUR PATH

First, you need to pick where to go on your hike. Ask an adult to help you look online for trails near you. Many parks have hiking trails.

Check to see if the path is easy or hard. How long is the trail? Is it flat or hilly? Make sure you are ready for the hike you choose.

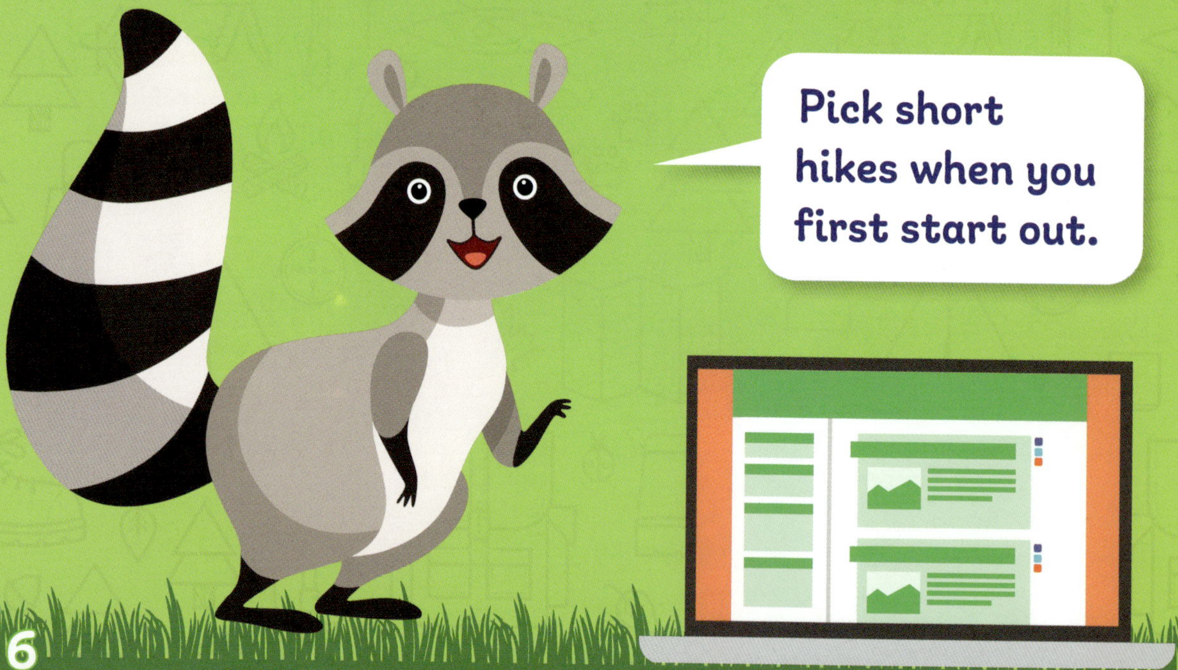

Pick short hikes when you first start out.

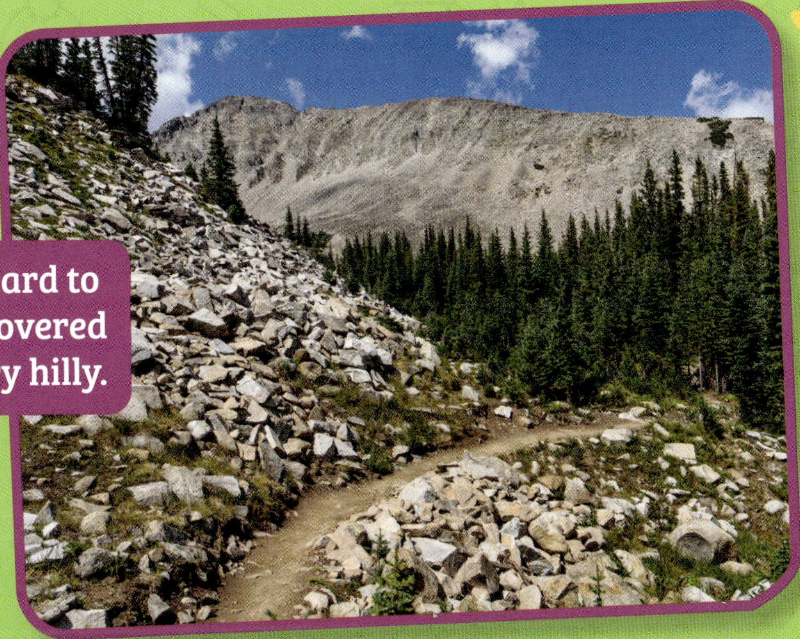

This trail might be hard to hike. The ground is covered in rocks, and it is very hilly.

The flat ground and even path may make this trail easier.

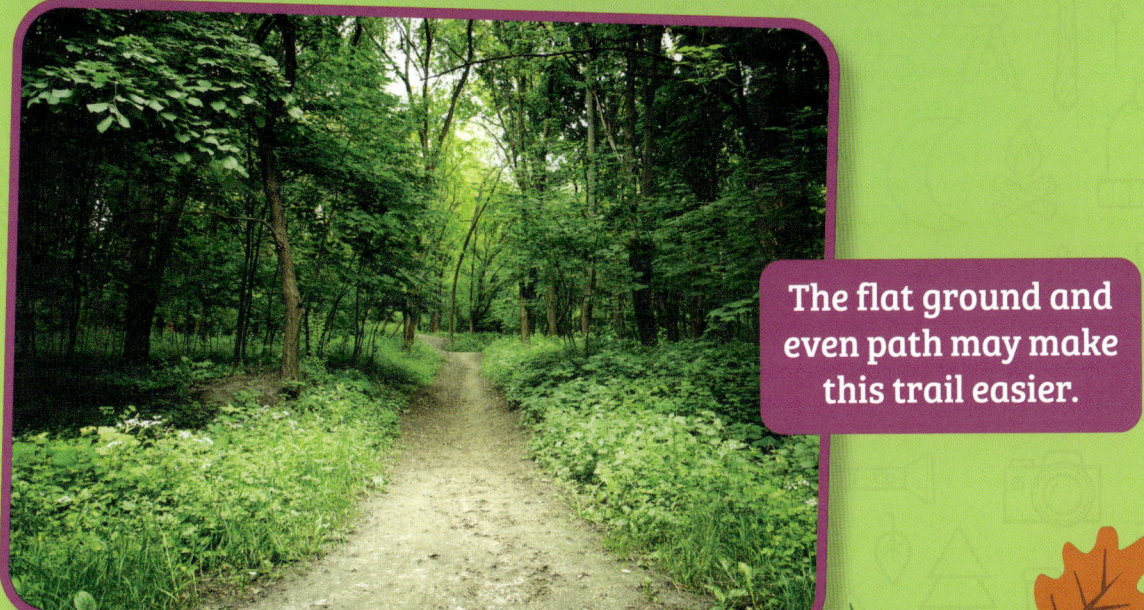

7

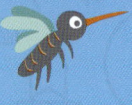

WHAT TO WEAR

What should you wear on your hike? You'll need sneakers or hiking boots. Closed-toed shoes like these keep your feet safe and help you stay **balanced**. Be sure to wear long, thick socks under your shoes.

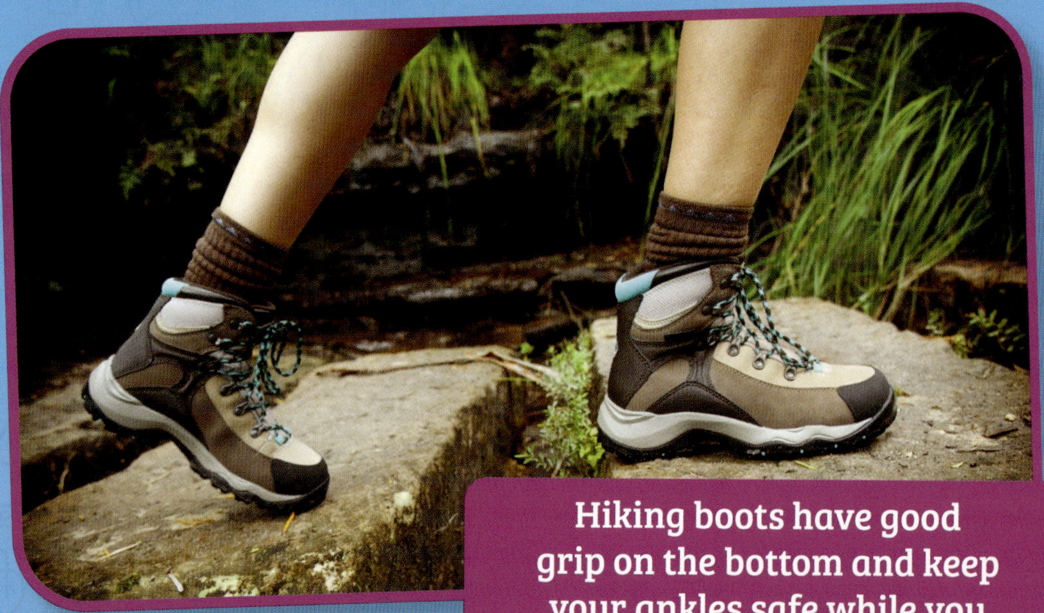

Hiking boots have good grip on the bottom and keep your ankles safe while you walk on uneven trails.

Wearing long sleeves and pants is a good idea, too. They **protect** you from bugs, scratchy branches, and the sun.

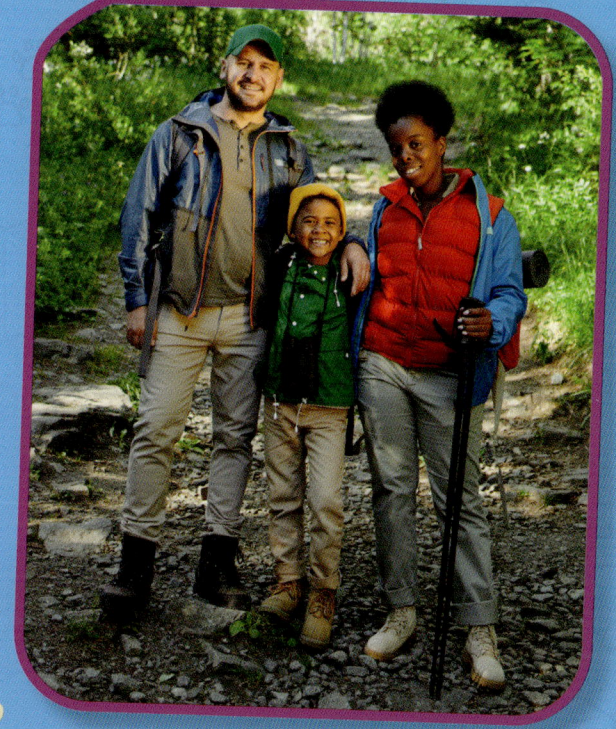

Bring a hat and sunscreen to be extra safe from the sun.

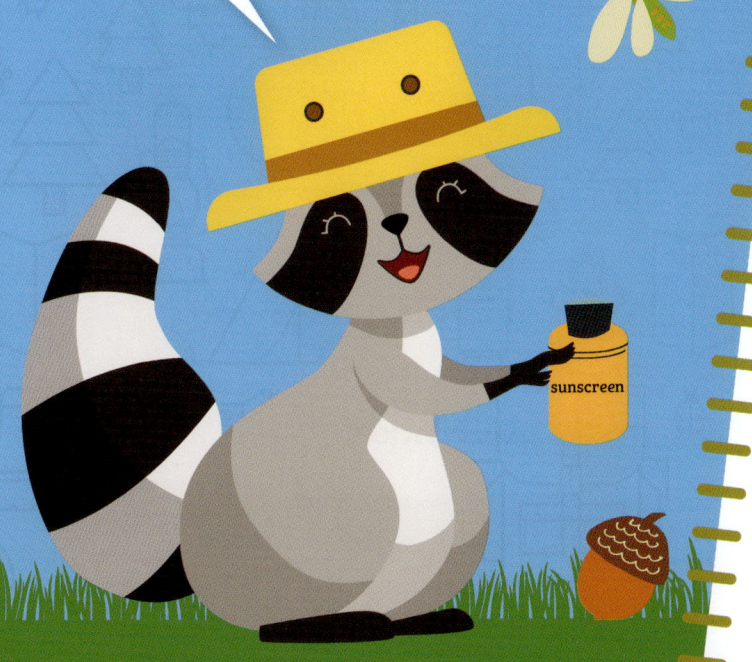

The weather can change fast while you are hiking. Dress in **layers** and think about bringing a raincoat.

FINDING YOUR WAY

Now it's time to gather the things you'll need for a day on the trail. What should you bring to make sure you don't get lost? A trail map shows you the different paths you can take.

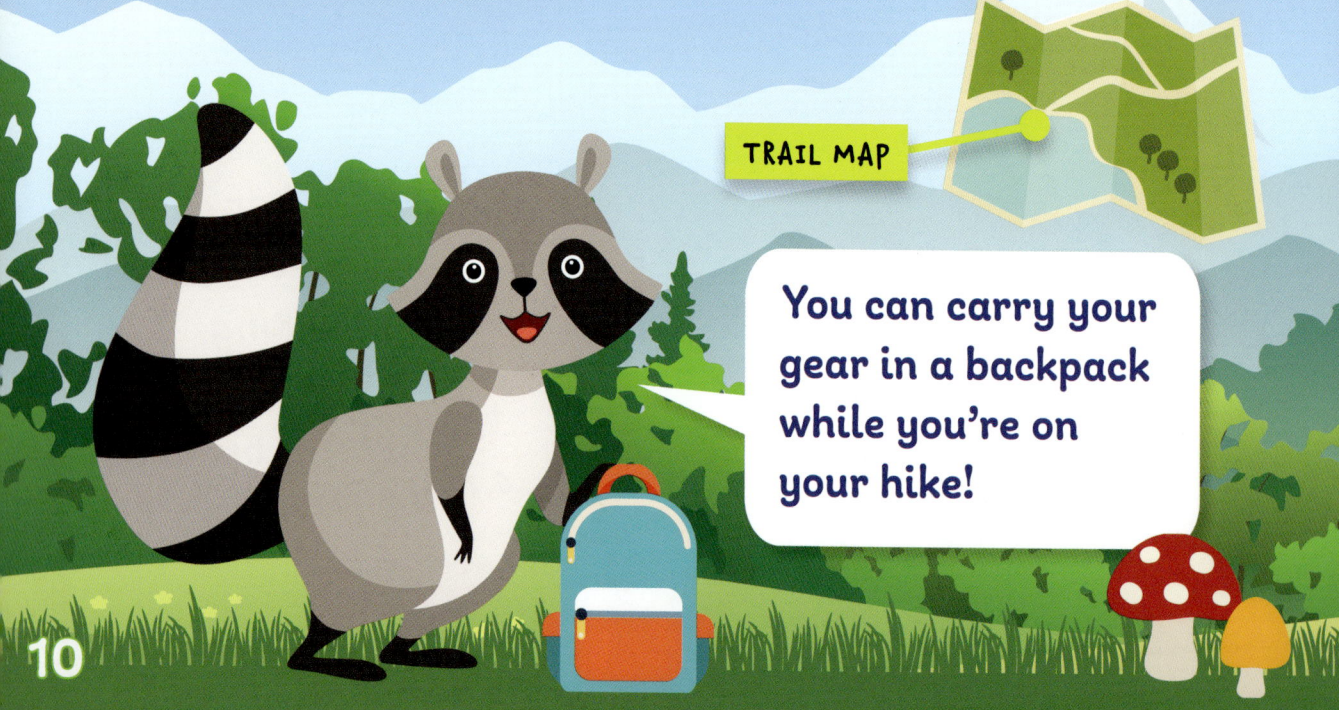

TRAIL MAP

You can carry your gear in a backpack while you're on your hike!

A compass helps you know which **direction** you are facing. To use it, turn the compass until the **needle** points north. Then, you can see all of the other directions, too.

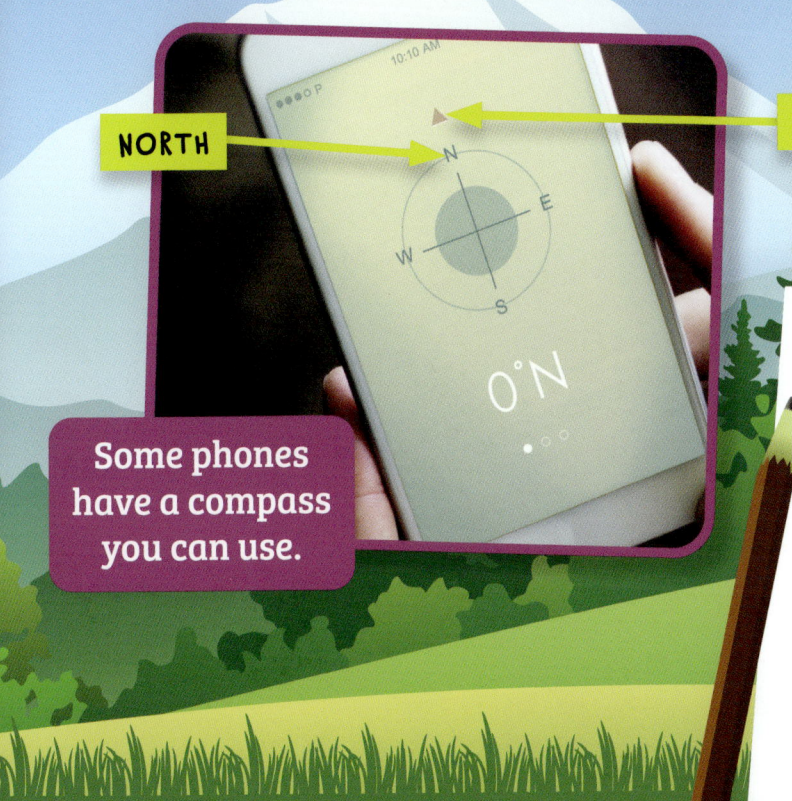

NORTH

NEEDLE

Some phones have a compass you can use.

Practice using your compass at home before you go hiking.

SAFETY GEAR

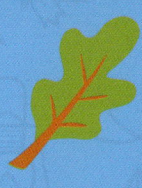

What else will you need? A walking stick can keep you balanced. It can also help you pull yourself up hills. You can use one to slow yourself as you go down hills, too.

Bring a **first aid kit** in your backpack. It can have small bandages to use in case you trip or fall.

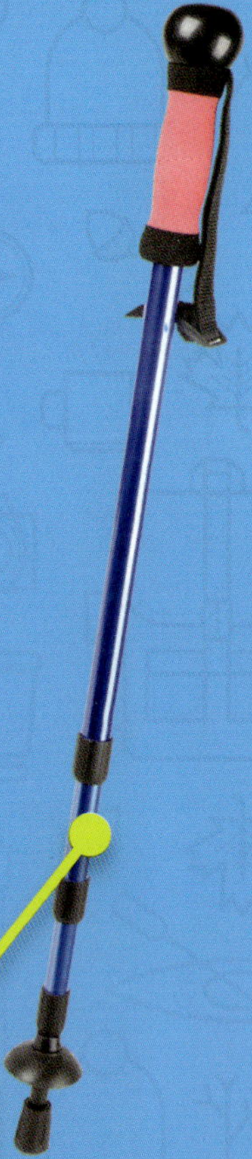

WALKING STICK

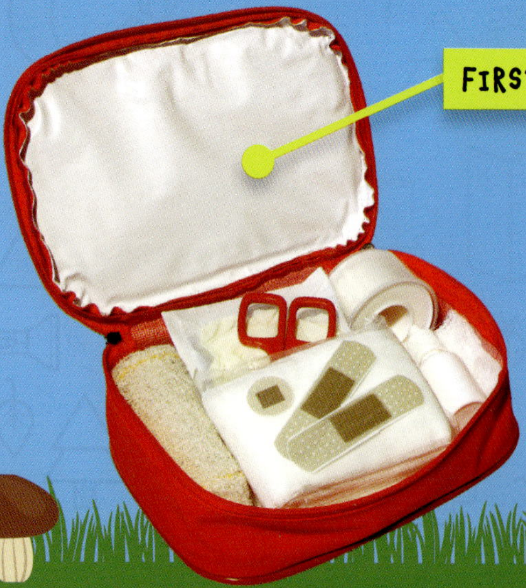

FIRST AID KIT

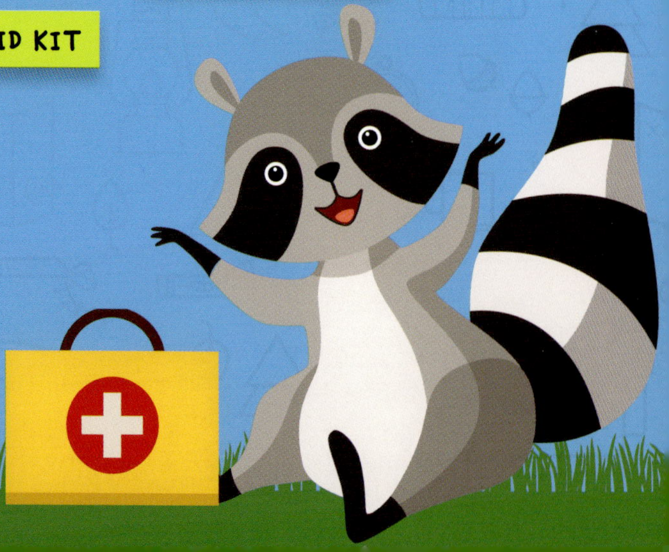

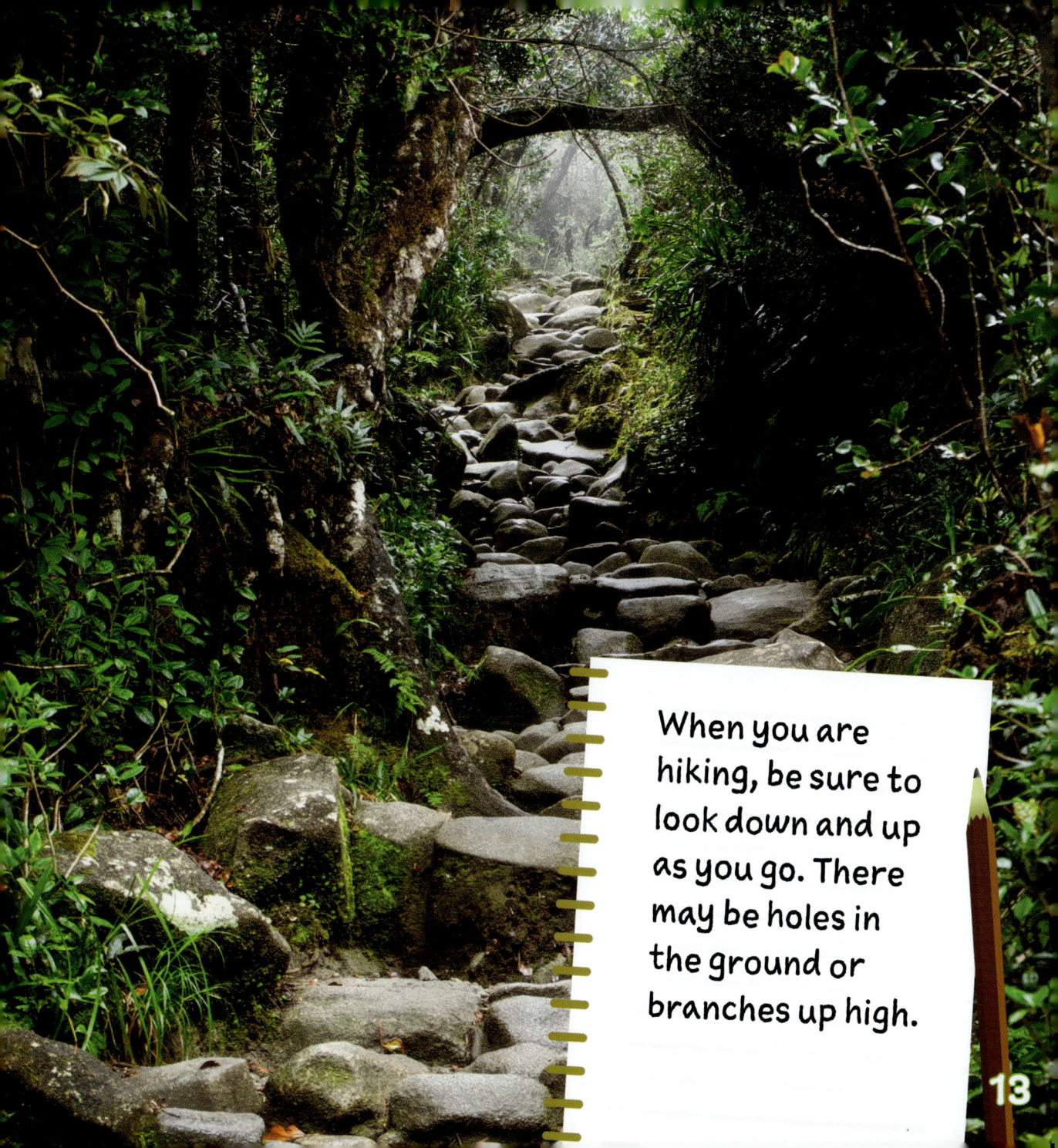

When you are hiking, be sure to look down and up as you go. There may be holes in the ground or branches up high.

HIKING SNACKS

Before you head out, be sure to pack some food. Hiking is hard work! It can make you hungry and thirsty. A healthy snack will give you **energy** to keep going.

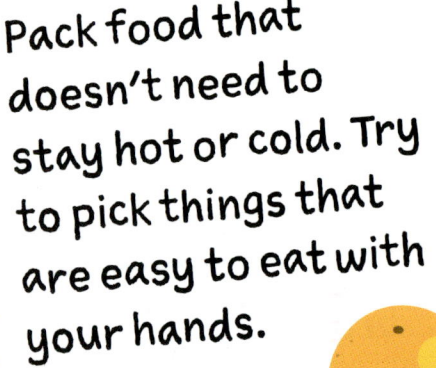

Pack food that doesn't need to stay hot or cold. Try to pick things that are easy to eat with your hands.

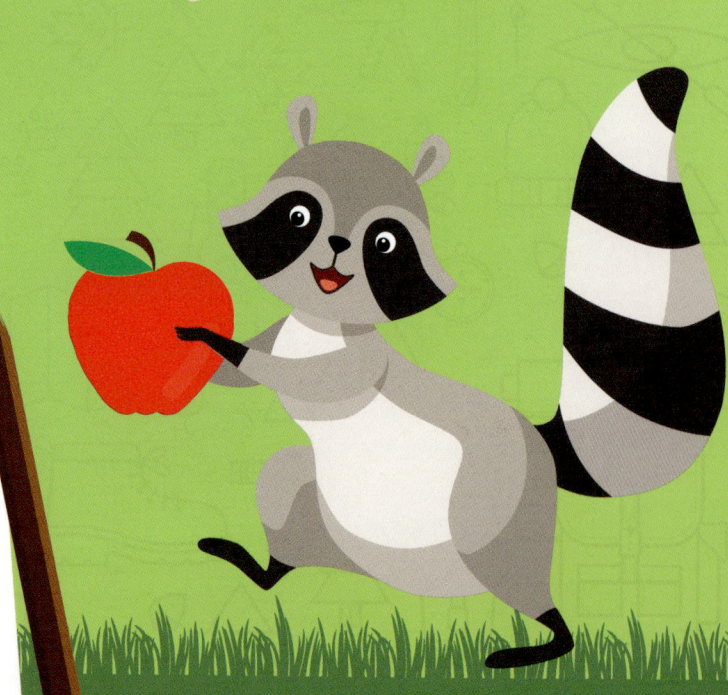

Water is very important when you hike. Bring a water bottle with you. If it's a hot day, you'll need even more water.

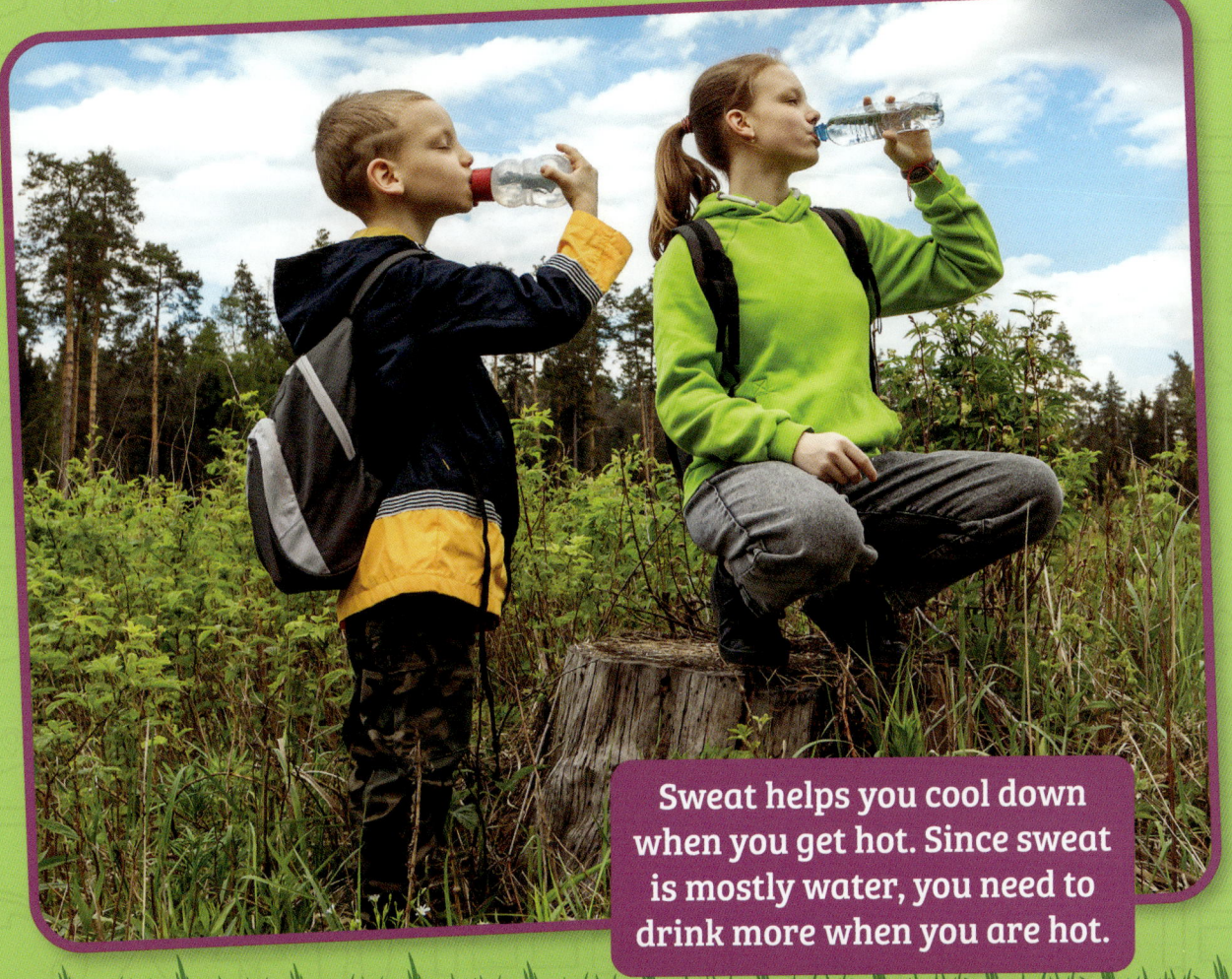

Sweat helps you cool down when you get hot. Since sweat is mostly water, you need to drink more when you are hot.

ON THE TRAIL

Now, gather your family or friends. It's time to explore! Just remember to follow some simple tips to share the trail.

When the path is narrow, walk in a single-file line. This makes room for other people using the trail.

There are more than 18,000 miles (29,000 km) of trails in the **National Park System**.

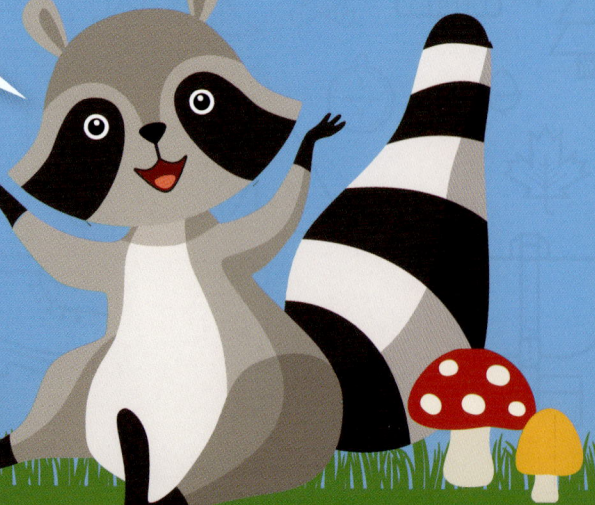

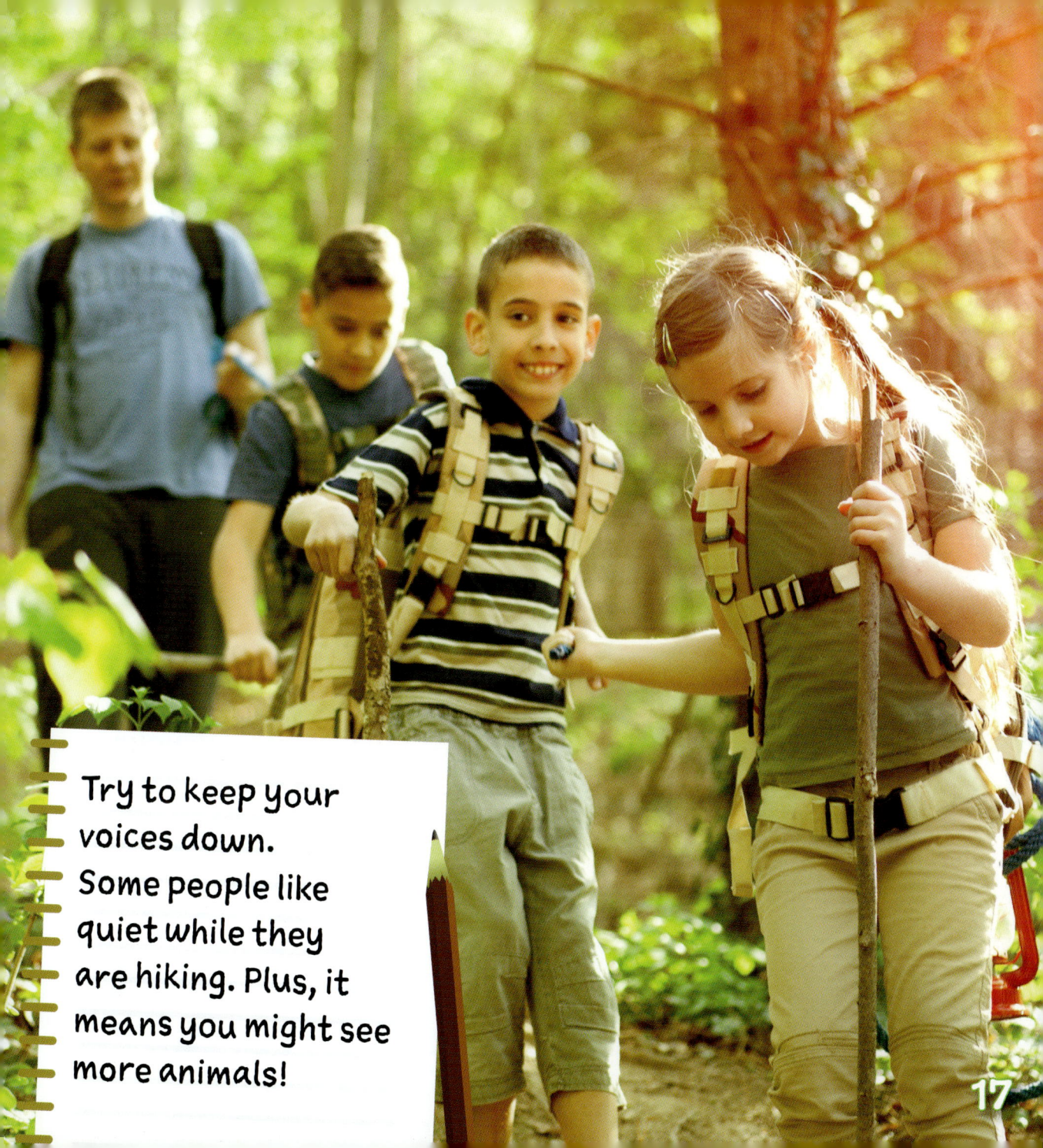

Try to keep your voices down. Some people like quiet while they are hiking. Plus, it means you might see more animals!

LIFE IN THE WILD

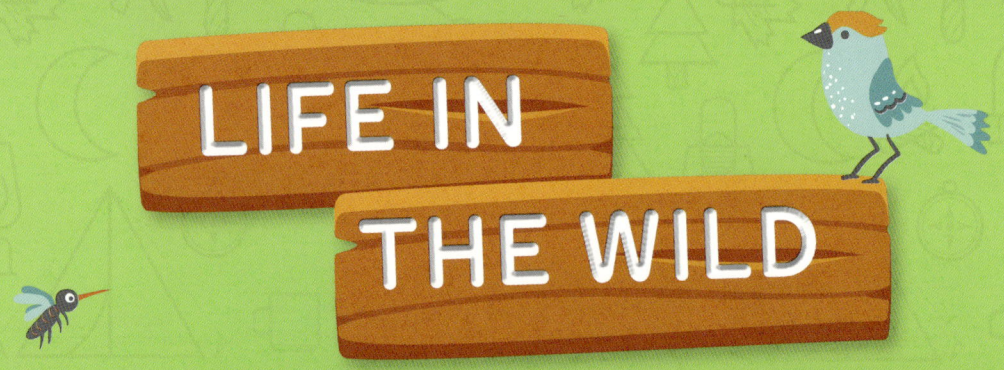

What will you see on your hike? You might spot some **wildlife.** Maybe you'll see birds, deer, or other animals. Always watch from a distance. Pick a hiking area far away from places where bears or mountain lions live.

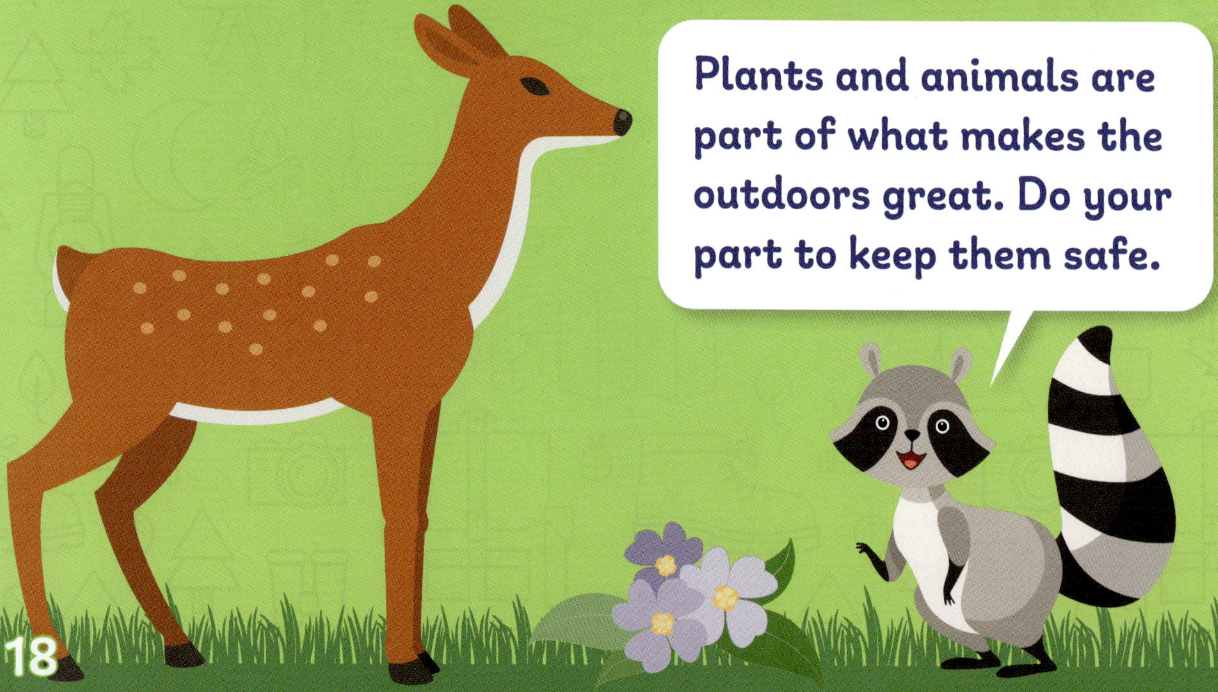

Plants and animals are part of what makes the outdoors great. Do your part to keep them safe.

Stay on the trail. Stepping on plants can hurt them. Little critters might make their homes just off the path, too.

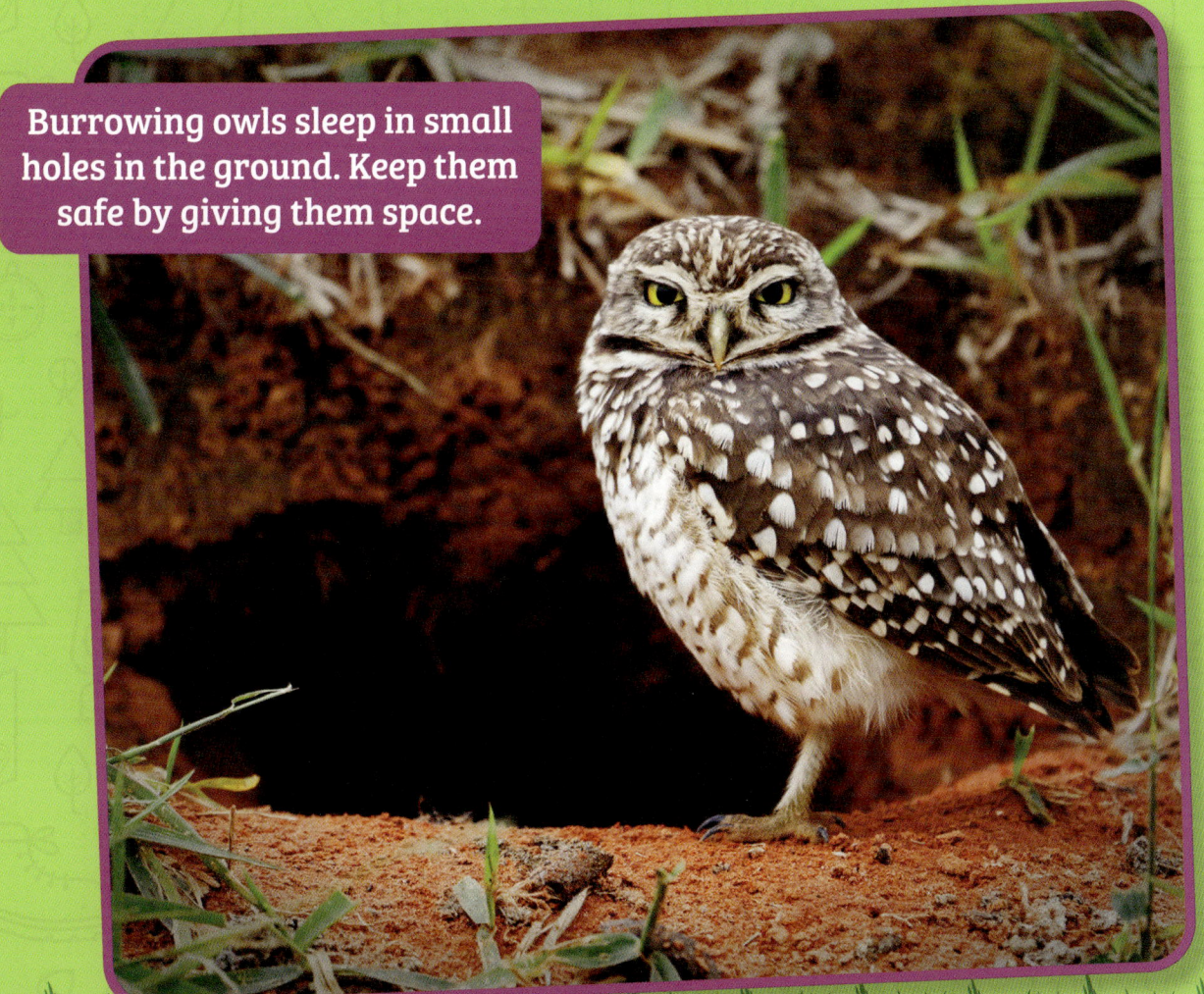

Burrowing owls sleep in small holes in the ground. Keep them safe by giving them space.

LEAVE NO TRACE

A good hiker follows the rule of leave no **trace**. This means you should leave plants or rocks the way you found them. Leave flowers for others to enjoy.

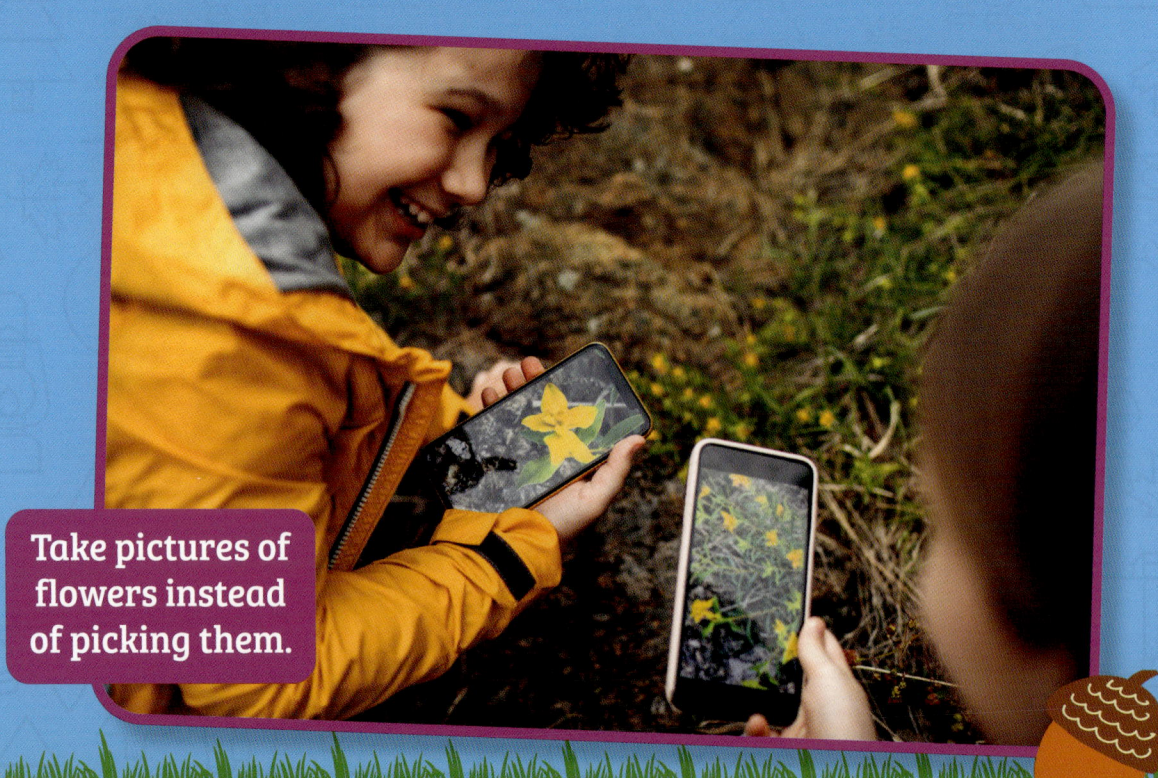

Take pictures of flowers instead of picking them.

This rule also means you should take your garbage with you. Make sure other people can also enjoy a beautiful hike free from your trash.

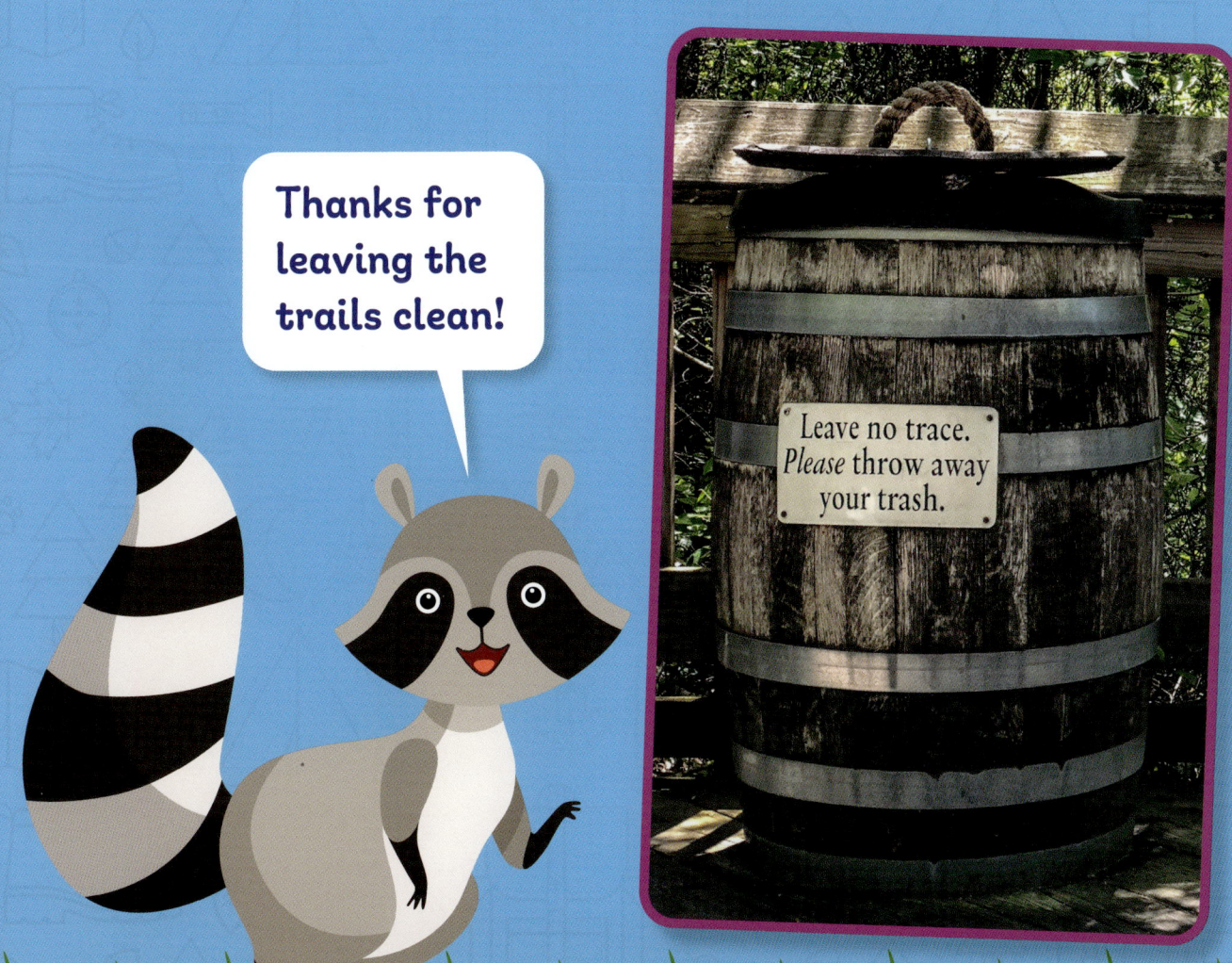

TAKE A HIKE

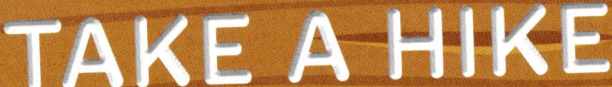

Hiking is a fun way to spend time outdoors! You can hike almost anywhere. Some trails lead through forests or fields. Others take you to the tops of mountains. You might pass lakes, rivers, or a waterfall. Every hike is a new adventure.

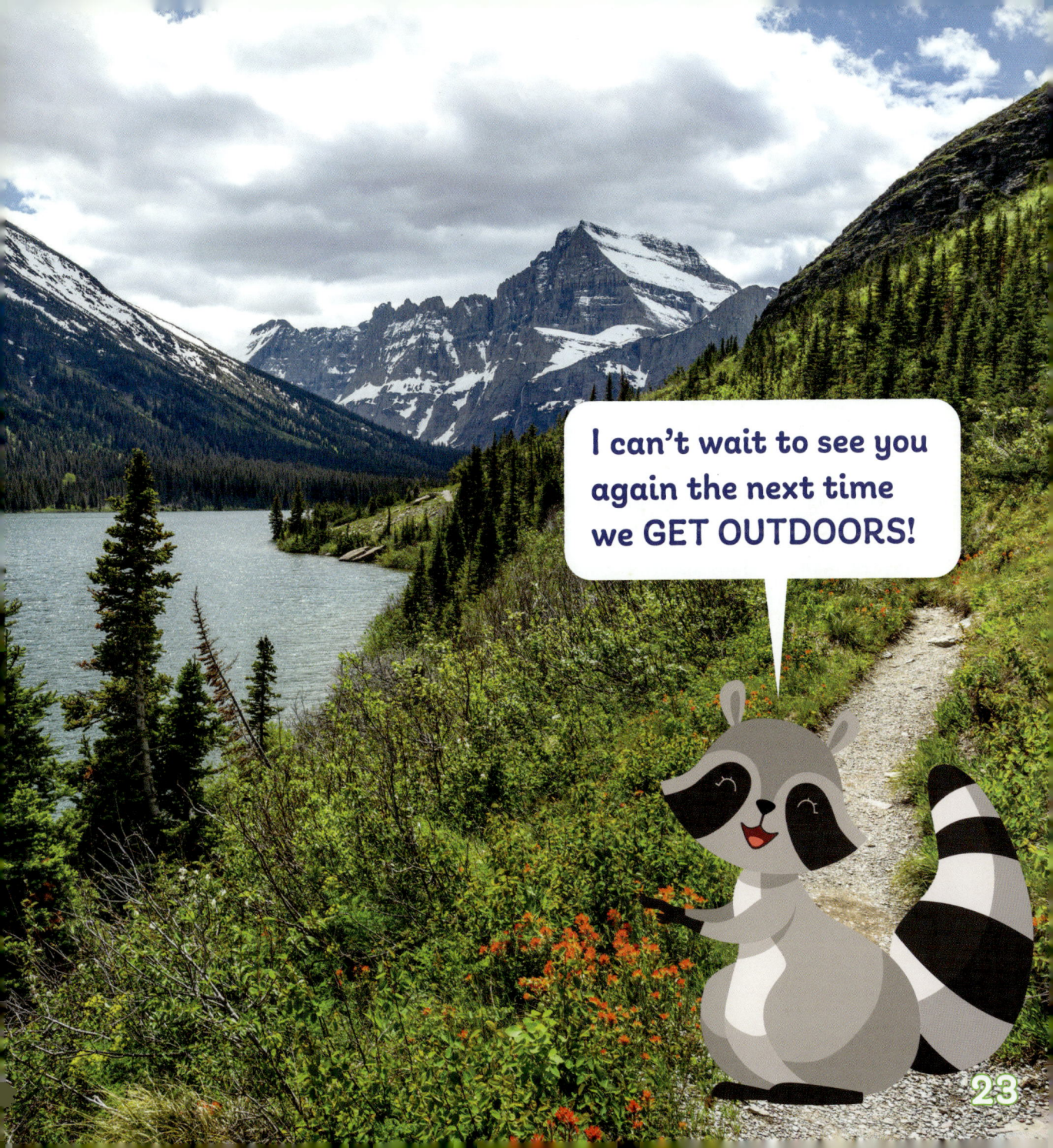

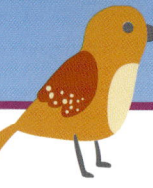

GLOSSARY

balanced upright and not in danger of losing control or falling

compass a tool used to find directions

direction one of the four main points of the compass, called north, south, east, or west

energy the power needed by all living things to grow and stay alive

first aid kit a box or bag of tools used to help people who are sick or injured

layers many levels of something, such as clothing, lying one over another

National Park System a group of parks that the U.S. government is in charge of

needle the small, thin piece of a compass that points

protect to keep safe from harm

trace a mark left by someone who has passed by

wildlife wild animals living in their natural setting

INDEX

animals 18–19
backpack 4, 10, 12
compass 4, 11
first aid kit 12
gear 10, 12
map 10
park 6, 16
walking stick 12
water 15
wildlife 18

DISCARD